5 Day Pouch Test Express Study Guide

Kaye Bailey

A LivingAfterWLS Publication
Volume 1: LivingAfterWLS Shorts

The 5 Day Pouch Test Express Study Guide
Find your weight loss surgery tool in five focused days.

Copyright © 2015 by Kaye Bailey; LivingAfterWLS, LLC.

5 Day Pouch Test Copyright © 2008, 2010, 2011, 2012, 2014, 2015 by Kaye Bailey and LivingAfterWLS, LLC. All rights reserved, including the right to reproduce this book or portions thereof in any form whatsoever. For information, address LivingAfterWLS, LLC, Post Office Box 311, Evanston, Wyoming 82931.

Health Advice: The health content in the 5 Day Pouch Test Express Study Guide is intended to inform, not prescribe, and is not meant to be a substitute for the advice and care of a qualified health-care professional. The author and publisher disclaim any liability arising directly or indirectly from the use of this book.

Nutritional Analysis: Every effort has been made to check the accuracy of the nutritional information that appears with each recipe. However, because numerous variables account for a wide range of values for certain foods, nutritive analyses in this book should be considered approximate. Different results may be obtained by using different nutrient databases and different brand-name products.

Published by
LivingAfterWLS, LLC
Post Office Box 311
Evanston, WY 82931

Printed by CreateSpace, An Amazon.com Company

COPYRIGHT © 2015 ~ ALL RIGHTS RESERVED
ISBN-13: 978-1518735967

CONTENTS

Welcome	Page 1
Plan Overview	Page 9
Days 1&2 Liquids	Page 19
Day 3 - Soft Protein	Page 27
Day 4 - Firm Proteins	Page 31
Day 5 - Solid Proteins	Page 35
FAQ's and Answers	Page 39
5DPT Recipes	Page 57

ONLY A TOOL

As owners of this powerful weight loss surgery tool we become stewards to work for it and work with it; to pursue our greatest potential through knowledge, practice, and personal responsibility.

WELCOME TO YOUR 5 DAY POUCH TEST EXPRESS STUDY GUIDE

Thank you for joining me in the 5 Day Pouch Test program and making it a valued tool in your weight loss surgery toolbox. In your hands is 5 Day Pouch Test Express Study Guide. This quick study provides the basics of the 5 Day Pouch Test plan to get you back on track with your weight loss or weight maintenance goals with weight loss surgery. For the comprehensive plan and complete tried and tested recipe collection get the 5 Day Pouch Test Owner's Manual.

What's in it: The Express Study Guide includes the plan summary broken down by day, 32 Frequently Asked Questions and Answers about the plan, and 10 sample recipes to get you started.

Who it's for: The 5 Day Pouch Test Express Study Guide is for those who want to learn a little more about the plan without investing in the manual; for people anxious to do the 5DPT and want a quick overview; for those who know the plan and have used it successfully who want a quick reference at their fingertips; people who want to succeed long term with their weight loss surgery tool.

Stay Connected: Subscribe to the 5 Day Pouch Test Bulletin delivered to your email Inbox. To receive our free monthly electronic newsletter, the "5 Day Pouch Test Bulletin", snap on the tag or visit 5DayPouchTest.com and enter your email address to subscribe. Also subscribe to our weekly "LivingAfterWLS Digest" and twice-monthly recipe newsletter, "Cooking with Kaye." We value and respect your online information: click the Privacy link on any of our web pages to learn more.

BROKEN WINDOWS HAPPEN.

There is a popular theory in urban renewal that suggests fixing broken windows as they happen is the key to reducing crime and preventing urban decay. George Kelling discusses the theory in a 1982 Atlantic Monthly article. He writes, "Consider a building with a few broken windows. If the windows are not repaired the tendency is for vandals to break a few more windows. Eventually, they may even break into the building, and if unoccupied, become squatters or cause destruction inside."

I believe it is possible to apply the "Broken Window" theory to our post-weight loss surgery health and wellness. The broken window, of course, would be a lapse in compliance with our program: eating unhealthy foods, the absence of exercise, and ignoring the rules. If we break a window one day and do not fix it the next then we risk breaking another window. But if we practice self-renewal and fix that broken window promptly we can avoid the intrusion of vandals and squatters who would break more windows and violate our bodies.

The challenge herein is that if we allow the broken window to go without repair we then become the vandals to our own body. At times it is far easier to give permission to the squatters than it is to evict them. One day of missed exercise leads to another and another and pretty soon the sloth-squatter has set-up camp in our building: our body. Over the holidays I missed several workout sessions and my sloth-squatter became quite at home enjoying free entry through my broken windows. When this happens immediate action must be taken to kick that squatter out. With determined self-renewal we must take control of our house.

Broken windows happen. In our homes and in our lives there will always be broken windows. A broken window is not a sign of failure or neglect. Windows are made of fragile glass that sometimes shatters. And though we may pretend to be tough as steel we are more like glass: fragile and prone to occasional breakage. Windows can be fixed. Let's fix our broken windows promptly and forbid the squatter's entry. We have worked hard for our new life. We deserve the gift of self-renewal.

The 5 Day Pouch Test will teach you to fix your broken windows. This is a highly structured back-to-basics five day plan that effectively repairs our broken windows and reminds us of the rules and guidelines that helped us use our tool to lose weight with surgery in the first place. The exclusive intent is not to lose weight: it is to get back-to-basics. Now is the time to repair our broken windows.

The 5 Day Pouch Test is most successful when we prepare mentally and emotionally to follow the plan as written and emerge on Day 6 enthusiastic to follow the Four Rules, make healthy food choices, exercise, and live well. The empowered feeling you get from completing the 5 Day Pouch Test will fuel a mental storm of enthusiasm similar to the excitement and can-do feelings you enjoyed during the early phase of weight loss following your surgical procedure.

SURGERY IS ONLY A TOOL

Surgery is only a tool. A tool is simply a device used to accomplish a task. Think of a carpenter at the workbench with his tools. Before the carpenter: a saw, a hammer, wood, a measuring stick and nails: all tools of the trade. The carpenter could stand before the tools and yearn for them to craft a magnificent treasure box. But the tools will not work on yearning alone. The carpenter must select the best tool for the task and then work with that tool using it to the best of his capability. The carpenter must work the tools.

And so it goes with our weight loss surgery tool. Yearning and desire will not cause the tool to craft the treasure of a healthy body. The tool will not work on hope alone.

As owners of this powerful weight loss surgery tool we become stewards to work for it, to pursue our greatest potential through knowledge, practice, and personal responsibility.

We must use the tool as a device to accomplish a task. If the tool breaks, such as a band slippage or failure, we must go to the repair shop for maintenance. The care of the tool is our responsibility. When we take responsibility for working the tool our chances for lasting success are great.

If we get comfortable in our post-weight loss surgery life there is a tendency to lose our determination. Perhaps we take it for granted. Maybe we just get bored or distracted. Maybe we get discouraged because life after surgery has been a struggle. Any of these things can cause us to lose hope or feel like failures. I have gone through periods of sadness and periods of euphoria since my weight loss surgery. Haven't you?

But just like we can work a plan to test the pouch, and work the tools, we can mentally train our mind to get back to being hell-bent determined to take personal control of our health. The 5 Day Pouch Test is the second step back to control. You have already taken the first step: seeking help. That is why you are here.

Now is the time to identify where you went off track. You will not be judged or made fun of. We all fall off track now and again. Be kind to yourself. A broken window is not a moral breakdown or personal failure; it is the product of living. Fixing the broken window is your responsibility. I am your champion in this cause.

You can do this!

Kaye

INTRODUCTION

Have you lost control of your weight loss surgery tool?

Does my pouch still work?

Have I broken my pouch?

Am I doomed to be a failure at this too?

Can I lose the weight I've regained?

Is the honeymoon period over?

I didn't make goal weight and now I'm gaining. Help!

If you are asking these questions then the 5 Day Pouch Test is for you. In 5 focused days you can rediscover your pouch, get back on track and lose weight with your weight loss surgery tool. You have not failed. You can learn to use the tool again.

This is the five day plan that I developed and use to determine if my pouch is working and return to that tight newbie feeling. And a bonus to this plan: it helps one get back to the basics of the weight loss surgery diet and in most cases it triggers weight loss. It is not difficult to follow and if you are in a stage of snacking and carb-cycling it will break this pattern. Sounds pretty good, right?

The 5 Day Pouch Test should never leave you feeling hungry. You can eat as much of the prescribed menu foods as you want during the day to satiate hunger and prevent snacking on slider foods and white carbs. You must drink a minimum of 64 ounces of water each day. The liquid restrictions (no liquids 30 minutes before or after meals and no liquid with meals) must be observed.

5DPT = 5 Day Pouch Test

Weight loss is not the exclusive intent of the 5 Day Pouch

Test. However, many who have completed this plan report a pleasing drop in weight. More importantly they celebrate a renewed sense of control over their pouch and eating habits. They easily transition back to a healthy post-surgical weight loss way of eating focused on lean-clean protein, vegetables, fruit, and limited dairy.

PLAN TO WORK THE PLAN

It sounds silly to offer a plan to work a plan but here I present a few ideas and hints for making the most of your 5DPT experience. The more prepared and enthused you are when you begin the 5DPT, the better your chances for success. Let's get started and let's get back on track!

Learn the plan. Read the plan in full and be sure you understand it. Read the plan completely in order to understand the progression of your diet from Day 1 to Day 5. Pay close attention to understanding the liquid restrictions and slider foods: these are the most common problem areas that lead to weight regain after weight loss surgery. As you become familiar with the 5 Day Pouch Test think back to how it compares with the early dietary stages following your weight loss surgery. Think back to what worked for you then and imagine the same will work for you again. Remember, you already know how to lose weight using your surgical tool. The effort you put into the 5DPT will return you to that place of healthy and reasonable weight management using your tool.

Remember: You already know how to use your surgical tool.

Mark the date. Set a date and mark your calendar. Make sure you can follow the plan without the disruption of travel, social events or hormonal cycles. Enlist the support of family and friends. It is fairly common for people to schedule the 5DPT to begin on Monday and end on Friday. But many have found that scheduling Day 1 for a Saturday works more favorably for them. On Days 1 and 2 one generally needs frequent bathroom breaks, which may be uncomfortable in a workplace. Consider that as you schedule your plan. Additionally, many of us have made the mistake of completing the 5DPT on Friday only to celebrate with weekend binge eating come Saturday. If our plan starts on Saturday and concludes on Wednesday we can more easily transition to a Day 6 lifestyle on Thursday, thus avoiding the weekend binge phenomena. Consider all of this before scheduling your 5 Day Pouch Test. Scheduling it for the right time significantly improves our chance for success.

Seek peer support. Decide who you will include in your plan and make known your expectations. Post to the Neighborhood or your online community asking for support from those who understand. The correct peer support nurtures our efforts in this recovery from relapse. We can learn from those who have traveled this path and tap into their enthusiasm. It is the nature of online support communities to cheer and celebrate each other's victories as well as buoy those who are struggling. Take advantage of this and gather your own cheering section to celebrate the baby steps that become big accomplishments. Become a support peer to others; when we are in this together: support of one another is symbiotic.

Make preparations. Plan your meals for all five days and do the grocery shopping before starting the 5DPT. We all know that the supermarket is temptation alley, do your best to avoid going there for these five days. An effective way to plan your meals is to use the 5 Day Pouch Test menu plan in Chapter 3. Make two copies of the 5DPT menu plan and use the first to plan your meals and snacks for all five days. This will become your shopping list as well as your map for the week. Many people are surprised at the relief and empowerment they feel upon making their food plan for five days. With the menu choices made there is little to dwell upon and we have spare energy to focus on getting back on track.

5DayPouchTest.com – Click on Tools

Mental readiness. Devote time to meditation focused on the 5 Day Pouch Test: why you are doing it and what you wish to accomplish. You practiced mental readiness before surgery and it served you well. Do the same now. You are about to embark on the repair process and exciting and good things will come to you for your initiative to take action. This is exciting stuff! Practice meditation your own way and build the excitement. If that means writing in a journal or listening to music or just spending quiet time thinking then do it. Mental readiness is essential in every life-endeavor worth taking.

Build your enthusiasm. The night before Day 1 create a storm of mental readiness by reading, discussing, and imagining your personal power to work the plan. Generate the same kind of excitement you had going into surgery. Go to bed empowered knowing you are about take control of the surgical tool you fought so hard to get in the first place.

THE 5 DAY POUCH TEST PLAN

This chapter presents the nuts and bolts of the 5 Day Pouch Test. Use this overview as a quick reference throughout the five days to keep track of where you are and where you are going.

5DPT: BRIEF OVERVIEW

It is only five days. And in the next five days you will learn your pouch is working; you will take control of your eating and snacking behaviors; and you will remember why you had weight loss surgery in the first place.

Days 1 and 2 of the plan are healing days. You treat your pouch like a newborn with gentle liquids and soups. Pouch inflammation is reduced and processed carbohydrate cravings subside. Mental focus is on listening to and respecting your body. Days 1 and 2 mimic the early days and weeks following bariatric surgery.

Day 3 introduces soft proteins like canned fish, fresh soft fish or eggs. This is the day we focus on tasting our food, chewing well, and enjoying the goodness of lean-clean protein. We focus on portion control and the liquid restrictions. On this day we start to remember what a tight pouch feels like and we appreciate the feeling of fullness.

Day 4 brings us to firm proteins like ground meat (beef, poultry, lamb, or game) and shellfish, scallops, lobster, salmon or halibut steaks. This is the day we truly realize the power of the pouch and most people are happily surprised to learn their pouch is not broken or stretched back to normal stomach size. The carbohydrate withdrawal is over, and energy levels are improving.

Day 5 finishes the test with solid proteins such as white meat poultry, beef steak, and any of the firm proteins from Day 4. The liquid restrictions are now a habit and we have successfully removed the slider foods from our diet. We have energy for exercise and for the daily tasks of living. Most importantly, we know our weight loss surgery tool works and we now have the confidence and capability to work the tool.

Day 6 is the way we will eat every day for the rest of our lives. Having successfully broken a carb-cycle, gained a feeling of control over the surgical gastric pouch, and possibly losing a few pounds one is ready for re-entry into a compliant way of eating. This means focusing on protein dense meals, observing the liquid restrictions, and avoiding starches, particularly processed carbohydrates and slider foods. Three meals a day should be two-thirds protein, one-third healthy carbohydrate in the form of low-glycemic vegetables and fruits. Consumption of whole grains is not forbidden, but should be limited to one serving a day.

BASIC TENETS ESSENTIAL TO SUCCESS

The following basic tenets are widely accepted by bariatric surgeons and nutritionists as lifestyle guidelines to be followed by people who have undergone all manner of gastric surgery for weight loss. I have found that making these tenets a lifestyle is the most effective way for me and many others to manage weight loss and maintain it with weight loss surgery. Refer to the documentation provided you at the time of your surgery for the specifics advised by your bariatric center. For our purposes each rule or tenet is summarized here for reference when learning and doing the 5 Day Pouch Test. Always keep in mind that we are doing the 5DPT to correct behavior and change trajectory so we may achieve different and more desirable results.

THE FOUR RULES OF WLS:
Protein First
Lots of Water
No Snacking
Daily Exercise

As patients we are well aware that WLS is frequently perceived by outsiders as an easy means to weight loss that requires little or no effort by the patient. It turns out there is nothing easy about the post-WLS lifestyle. At the time of surgery we agreed to follow Four Rules of dietary and lifestyle management guidelines for the rest of our life in order to lose weight and maintain a healthy weight. This is our burden and our responsibility if we wish to keep morbid obesity in remission.

THE FOUR RULES

All surgical weight loss procedures including gastric bypass, adjustable gastric banding (lap-band) and gastric sleeve, promote weight loss by decreasing energy (caloric) intake with a reduced or restricted stomach size. The small stomach pouch is only effective when a patient rigorously follows the Four Rules: eat a high protein diet; drink lots of water; avoid snacking on empty calorie food; engage in daily exercise.

In our introduction to a bariatric program we were taught and agreed to follow the standard Four Rules which work in concert with our surgically altered stomach and digestive system to bring about rapid massive weight loss. In fact, most of us were asked during the psychological evaluation if we could commit to following the Four Rules. Like me, I bet you said "Of course" with complete confidence. What I missed in the orientation was that these rules would be a way of life for the rest of my life. Let's take a quick look at each rule as it applies to WLS patients.

Protein First: At every meal the WLS patient will eat lean animal, dairy, or vegetable protein before any other food. Protein shakes or supplements may be included as part of the weight loss surgery diet. Patients are advised to consume 60-105 grams of protein a day. Eating lean protein will create a tight feeling in the surgical stomach pouch: this feeling is the signal to stop eating. Many patients report discomfort when eating lean protein, yet this discomfort is the very reason the stomach pouch is effective in reducing food and caloric intake. Animal products are the most nutrient rich source of protein and include fish, shellfish, poultry, and meat. Dairy protein, including eggs, yogurt, and cheese, is another excellent source of protein.

Lots of Water: Like most weight loss programs, bariatric surgery patients are instructed to drink lots of water throughout the day. Most centers advise a minimum of 64 fluid ounces of water each day. Water hydrates the organs and cells and facilitates the metabolic processes of human life. Water flushes toxins and waste from the body. Patients are strongly discouraged from drinking carbonated beverages. In addition, patients are warned against excessive alcohol intake as it tends to have a quicker and more profound intoxicating affect compared with pre-surgery consumption. In addition, non-nutritional beverages of any kind may lead to weight gain and increased snacking.

No Snacking: Patients are discouraged from snacking which may impede weight loss and lead to weight gain. Specifically, patients are forbidden to partake of traditional processed carbohydrate snacks, such as chips, crackers, baked goods, and sweets. Patients who return to snacking on empty calorie non-nutritional food defeat the restrictive nature of the surgery and weight gain results. It is seemingly contradictory that the 5DPT allows snacking. High protein snacks are allowed because they keep the metabolism active, they satiate hunger, and they help relieve the symptoms of carbohydrate withdrawal.

Daily Exercise: In general patients are advised to engage in 30 minutes of physical activity on most days of the week. The most effective way to heal the body from the ravages of obesity is to exercise. Exercise means moving the body: walking, stretching, bending, inhaling and exhaling. Exercise is the most effective, most enjoyable, most beneficial gift one can receive when recovering from life threatening, crippling morbid obesity. Consistent exercise will keep morbid obesity in remission and help compensate for lapses in following the three other rules. People who successfully maintain their weight exercise daily.

SLIDER FOODS & LIQUID RESTRICTIONS

Slider Foods: To the weight loss surgery patient slider foods are the bane of good intentions often causing dumping syndrome, weight loss plateaus, and eventually weight gain. By definition slider foods are soft simple processed carbohydrates of little or no nutritional value that slide right through the surgical stomach pouch without providing nutrition or satiation. The most commonly consumed slider foods include pretzels, crackers (saltines, graham, Ritz®, etc.) filled cracker snacks such as Ritz Bits®, popcorn, cheese snacks (Cheetos®) or cheese crackers, tortilla chips with salsa, potato chips, sugar-free cookies, cakes, and candy.

The very nature of the surgical gastric pouch is to cause feelings of tightness or restriction when one has eaten enough food. However, when soft simple carbohydrates are eaten this tightness or restriction does not result and one can continue to eat, unmeasured amounts of food without ever feeling uncomfortable. Many patients unknowingly turn to slider foods for this very reason. They do not like the discomfort that results when the pouch is full from eating a measured portion of lean animal or dairy protein, and it is more comfortable to eat the soft slider foods. Slider foods have played a significant role in every case of post-WLS weight regain that I have ever heard about.

Liquid restrictions: After surgical weight loss patients are advised to avoid drinking liquids 30 minutes before meals and 30 minutes after meals. (The time restriction varies from surgeon to surgeon, but most use the 30 minutes before, 30 minutes after restriction. Follow your surgeon's specific directions.) In addition there should be no liquid consumed while eating. Following these liquid restrictions allows the pouch to feel tight sooner and stay tight longer, thus leaving the patient feeling satiated for greater periods of time without experiencing the urge to snack. In addition, the longer food stays in the small gastric pouch the more opportunity the body has to absorb nutrients from that food. The liquid restrictions should be followed when eating all meals and snacks, including protein shakes, protein bars, hearty soups, and solid protein main dishes.

Gentle reminder: This is not about perfection

I have never done the 5DPT perfectly and I do not know anyone that has. Rather than make the five days about perfection make this time about learning. Little mistakes will not stop the world from turning. So forge ahead doing your very best and forgive little mistakes. Learn from each day, make notes on your 5 Day Pouch Test Journal (download at 5DayPouchTest.com click Tools), and emerge on Day 6 knowing more about yourself and how to work your tool.

If we complete the 5 Day Pouch Test having learned a few things about our self, our weight loss surgery and our capability in managing life and weight loss surgery in relationship to one another we have succeeded: we can deem the 5 Day Pouch Test a success. Here are some things to consider while embracing the 5DPT as a learning experience:

PLAN YOUR 5 DAY POUCH TEST MENU

One of the best ways to enable your success with the 5 Day Pouch Test is to plan in advance your meals for the duration of the plan. This is not a difficult task as you are only planning for five days. Many find having a complete plan to be liberating: the decision making is done. One must only concentrate on following the plan and focusing on surgical pouch and how it functions when used properly. Here are some helpful suggestions for planning your 5DPT menu:

For each day plan three meals (breakfast, lunch, dinner) and two or three snacks. Foods from Days 1 and 2 may be advanced to Days 3, 4, and 5. Do not bring foods from Days 3, 4, and 5 back to Days 1 and 2.

Purchase and store groceries for the 5DPT before Day 1 and avoid going to the market during the five days. The 5DPT will help build your resistance to marketing temptation, but during the five days the temptation may simply be an annoying distraction.

If you haven't tried protein gelatin or protein pudding before make a sample before your 5DPT. Make certain that what you plan is something you will enjoy eating. Consider 1-cup servings of soup as a suitable snack on any day of the 5DPT.

If including soups on Days 1 and 2 prepare them in advance before Day 1 and divide into 1-cup serving containers for ease of use.

All of the 5DPT recipes are healthy and family friendly. Try to include the people at your table in your menu and avoid cooking two meals. For others add vegetables, a salad or a starch as desired.

Try to stick with your menu plan as closely as possible. Sometimes change is unavoidable. Do the best you can at each meal staying as close to your plan as possible.

THE REAL WORLD

Develop strategies for navigating in the real world. When we have surgery we changed and then we returned to the exact environment we lived in prior to surgery: the very environment that contributed to our obesity. The only chance we have to make the surgery work is to evolve strategies for navigating our new body in the old waters.

MY PLANNING NOTES:

SAMPLE 5 DAY POUCH TEST MENU

Day 1:
Breakfast: Choco-Mocha Morning Smoothie
Morning Snack: High-Protein Gelatin or 1 small orange
Lunch: Vanilla-Berry Smoothie
Afternoon Snack: 1/2 apple
Dinner: 1 cup 5DPT soup of your Choice
Evening Snack: High Protein Pudding

Day 2:
Breakfast: Choco-Mocha Morning Smoothie
Morning Snack: Frozen Protein Pudding Pop
Lunch: 1 cup 5DPT soup of your choice
Afternoon Snack: High Protein Gelatin
Dinner: 1 cup 5DPT soup of your Choice
Evening Snack: High Protein Pudding

Day 3:
Breakfast: Mock Breakfast Burrito
Morning Snack: High Protein Gelatin
Lunch: Parmesan Tuna Patty
Afternoon Snack: Frozen Protein Pudding Pop
Dinner: Parmesan Tuna Patty
Evening Snack: High Protein Gelatin

Day 4:
Breakfast: Spinach-Sausage Egg Bake
Morning Snack: 1 small orange
Lunch: Parmesan Tuna Patty (leftover from Day 3)
Afternoon Snack: 1 small pear and 1/2 cup cottage cheese
Dinner: Orange Glazed Salmon
Evening Snack: High Protein Pudding

Day 5:
Breakfast: Egg Brunch Bake
Morning Snack: 1 piece of low-glycemic fruit
Lunch: Orange Glazed Salmon (leftover from Day 4)
Afternoon Snack: High Protein Gelatin
Dinner: Chicken and Pea Pods
Evening Snack: Frozen Protein Pudding Pop

MAKE A PLAN, NOT A WISH

"Simply not wanting to be overweight is a wish, not a plan. One way to motivate yourself is to recognize how gratifying it is to make a commitment to a goal, identify the specific steps to get there, follow your plan, and reap the rewards."
(Judith J. Wurtman & Nina Frusztajer Marquis, 2006)

MY MENU PLAN:

DAYS 1 & 2 - LIQUIDS

Days 1 and 2 of the plan are healing days. You treat your pouch like a newborn with gentle liquids and soups. Pouch inflammation is reduced and processed carbohydrate cravings subside. Mental focus is on listening to and respecting your body. Your menu on Days 1 and 2 mimics the early days and weeks following bariatric surgery. A diet of simple liquids, including protein drinks, clear broth, creamy soups, and hearty soups takes the guess work out of meal planning so you can focus on making well and making right your WLS tool.

All meals on Days 1 and 2 are liquids as defined here. In the 5 Day Pouch Test liquids are defined to include clear broth and creamy soups, protein fortified beverages (protein shakes), and hearty soups made of vegetables, legumes with some animal protein and dairy. See the recipe section for delicious and healthy recipes to enjoy on Days 1 and 2. Many people find that including both protein fortified meal replacement shakes and the hearty soups in their diet on Days 1 and 2 improves their overall experience with the 5DPT. The purpose of all liquids is to disrupt snacking, grazing, or processed carbohydrate eating habits. In addition, the liquids will work to soothe and cleanse your system and prepare you for the following three days.

> Liquids are defined to include clear broth and creamy soups, protein fortified beverages, and hearty soups made of vegetables, legumes, and some animal protein and dairy.

Do not restrict food or caloric intake on the 5DPT

You can have as many liquid meals as needed in response to hunger or cravings. Some people are inclined to restrict food intake during the 5 Day Pouch Test: this is not encouraged because it leads to increased hunger cravings and frustration. Do not restrict food intake: less is not better. Pay close attention to the signals your body gives and when you are hungry eat something from the approved menu for the day. Soups are measured in 1-cup servings and protein drinks are measured as the recipe or package directs. Stick with these portion sizes and eat what you can in 15 minutes. After 15 minutes discard what is uneaten and take pause to experience your pouch noting feelings of fullness and satiation. Wait at least one full hour before your next serving of liquid meal. Use this time to be mindful of your body; to get in touch with your pouch. Learning to feel the pouch and listening for authentic biological hunger signals is essential to your successful weight management. If you are truly hungry after waiting one hour then have another serving of one of the approved meals.

Time all meals: 15 minutes

Many bariatric centers recommend patients take 30 minutes to eat meals. Some even instruct patients to use a stopwatch and time three minutes between bites of food. The reason is to slow down the eating habits of the recovering morbidly obese person. As the patient recovers from surgery and becomes more comfortable eating they tend to eat more volume and often continue to eat over the 30 minutes allowed for a meal, even though satiation has already been achieved. Eventually the caloric intake at meals increases in spite of the stomach pouch restrictions. This is particularly true for patients who introduce beverages back into their meal disregarding the liquid restrictions.

During the pouch test a person is following the liquid restrictions and eating a high protein diet. By limiting meal time to 15 minutes one will enjoy the satisfying feeling that is the desired result of a gastric pouch.

The following is from the Gastric Bypass Instructions from Alvarado Hospital:

"When you feel satisfied you are finished. Don't get trapped in the belief that you have to eat everything on your plate, or that you can't possibly get by with that small a meal. Your meals will be small, and they are supposed to be small. If you feel full and satisfied and you try to eat any more you will begin to feel nauseated; and you may throw up. The point is not to see how close you can come to nausea. Learn to eat until satisfied and to avoid getting sick." *(Wittgrove 1999)*

UNDERSTANDING THE LIQUID OPTIONS

Protein Fortified Beverages: Protein shakes, protein drinks, protein breakfast drinks are all protein fortified beverages. Look for ready-to-drink (RTD) beverages that have at least 15 grams of protein and fewer than 5 grams of carbohydrate per serving. Protein powder drinks are acceptable as well, providing they meet the same criterion of 15 grams protein and fewer than 5 grams carbohydrate. Homemade protein smoothies are a favorable addition to the 5DPT menu. They can be created with or without protein powder using low-fat cottage cheese, yogurt and fruit or berries. See the recipe section. Each of us has a unique taste preference when it comes to protein beverages. You are responsible for finding the protein beverage you like and using it as part of your long-term weight management diet.

Clear broth or creamy soups: Clear broth and creamy soups are a favorite comfort food for many of us. Canned commercial chicken broth, beef broth, and vegetable broth are enjoyable meals on Days 1 and 2. Look for ready-to-eat broth that is low-sodium or reduced sodium and enjoy 1-cup servings. Do not drink any liquids for 30 minutes before or after having a warm cup of broth. Again, we want the pouch to absorb the nutrients from the food and we want to feel full as long as possible. Even though clear broth is a liquid of similar viscosity to water it contains nutrients and energy from which the body benefits.

Swanson ready-to-eat 50% Less Sodium Beef Broth® is a good example of readily available commercial clear soup appropriate for the 5DPT. A 1-cup serving provides 15 calories, 3 grams protein, 1 grams carbohydrate, no fat and 400mg sodium. When shopping for a commercial soup, look for nutritional data that is comparable to this example. There are many good regional soups available at specialty food stores and larger supermarkets. Do some exploring and find something you can enjoy knowing you are feeding your body well.

A quality protein powder will add as many as 21 grams of protein to your 1-cup serving of soup. Tip: When you find a protein powder you like try including it in your meals as often as possible. Good quality protein supplementation is a terrific tool in our ongoing weight management strategy.

Creamy soups are a comfort food favorite for Days 1 and 2. Many creamy soups include dairy products such as milk, cream, sour cream, or half-and-half. For purposes of the 5DPT full-fat dairy should be used as called for in the Day 1 and 2 recipes because it improves satiation longer than no-fat or reduced fat food. Note: After the 5DPT feel free to modify the soups with reduced or low-fat dairy as you find appropriate with your ongoing weight management. The soups are very good and always a welcome inclusion in a healthy Day 6 and beyond diet. People with lactose intolerance should avoid including creamy soups in their 5DPT and their regular diet. Select the hearty soups or clear broths instead.

Campbell's Healthy Request® Cream of Mushroom Soup is a good commercial soup that works well on the 5DPT. A 1-cup serving of soup prepared with 2% milk provides 130 calories, 6 grams protein, 5 grams fat (1 gram saturated), 10 grams carbohydrate, and 410mg sodium. For on-the-go meals try Campbell's Soup at Hand® 25% Less Sodium Classic Tomato Soup. Heated quickly in the microwave and served in the same container this convenient soup provides 140 calories, 3g protein, 0g fat, 33g carbohydrate and 480mg sodium. Use these examples to find ready-to-eat creamy soups you will enjoy including in your 5DPT and beyond.

Hearty Soups: As I developed this plan I learned that more substantial soups made of animal protein, legumes, beans, and low-glycemic vegetables work well to alleviate the discomfort and stress of a liquid diet. These satisfying soup recipes are made of foods low on the Glycemic Index (GI), a measure of how your blood glucose levels are affected by food. That means they will stick with you without causing a rapid rise and subsequent drop in blood glucose. These great comfort soups will help keep you feeling full longer, help you achieve and maintain a healthy weight, and provide you with more consistent energy throughout the day.

When including hearty soups as part of your 5DPT menu I encourage you to cook and enjoy the recipes provided. These recipes are specific to the plan and they work very well in our five day dietary progression. An added bonus: the soup recipes offered are less expensive per serving than prepared soups or protein drinks and they are family friendly making the 5 Day Pouch Test practical to incorporate into our busy schedules. Check out the recipe section for delicious soups and smoothies and make them a part of your LivingAfterWLS way of life.

Soups vs. Sliders: It is easy to confuse soup with slider foods since both are liquids that flow more rapidly through the stoma than solid protein. Remember, the soup recipes provided are nutrient dense. Slider foods by definition, are non-nutritional and non-filling. In addition, when we enjoy soup and observe the liquid restrictions our body benefits from the vitamins and nutrients in the meal while we enjoy a comforting feeling of satiation.

CARBOHYDRATE WITHDRAWAL

Carbohydrate withdrawal: When any heavily consumed food is withdrawn from the diet the body is likely to experience symptoms of withdrawal that may include headache, dizziness, cramping, and nausea. This is not unique to our WLS body; this is a simple fact of biology. On the 5DPT when processed carbs are withdrawn many people report symptoms of "carbohydrate withdrawal." Do not suffer through this. If you notice symptoms of carbohydrate withdrawal eat a small piece of melon, some berries, an apple or an orange. Any low-glycemic fruit or vegetable will reduce the symptoms of carbohydrate withdrawal.

You may also try a serving of Emergen-C® energy booster fizzy drink mix, which is known to reduce the symptoms and discomfort of carbohydrate withdrawal. In addition, Emergen-C® provides B vitamins for energy and C vitamins for immunity along with many other vitamins and minerals. You can count a serving of Emergen-C® as part of your daily intake of water. Do not be put off by the 5 or 6 grams carbohydrate per serving: these are beneficial nutrient dense big-bang-for-your-buck carbs. Enjoy!

For nausea, try sipping freshly brewed warm green tea or ginger herbal tea. You can add fresh ginger juice to further ease the symptoms of stomach distress and nausea.

DAYS 1 & 2 KEY LEARNING POINTS

Heal your pouch with soothing comforting liquids that are nutrient dense and low glycemic.

Time your meals: 15 minutes per meal.

Make informed dietary choices when eating at home, commercially prepared food or eating out.

Do not suffer through carbohydrate withdrawal. Low glycemic fruits and vegetables reduce discomfort. Also try herbal tea or Emergen-C®.

Revisit the empowerment you enjoyed after surgery: you are a powerful and capable person and you are getting back on track!

MY NOTES DAYS 1 & 2:

RECIPE FOR SUCCESS:

Please follow the 5DPT as it is written: it was developed to help you achieve the best results with your weight loss surgery. We tested it numerous times so you don't have to.

DAY 3 - SOFT PROTEIN

As on Days 1 and 2, for the next three days you get to eat as much as you want as often as you want. But there is a catch: you must follow the plan. Again there are specific menu choices for Day 3. Today we introduce soft protein served in carefully measured portions. After two days of 5DPT liquids the introduction of soft protein is a welcome dietary change. It is likely on Day 3 you will start to feel that "newbie" tightness in your pouch. In addition, your hunger or carb cravings are likely to be diminished. Continue to observe the liquid restrictions and take your meals only on a "dry" pouch. Your dry pouch will hold soft protein longer prolonging feelings of satiety.

Protein Recommendations Day 3: canned fish (tuna or salmon) mixed with lemon and seasoned with salt and pepper, eggs cooked as desired seasoned with salt pepper and/or salsa, fresh soft fish (tilapia, sole, orange roughy), baked or grilled, and lightly seasoned. Yogurt and cottage cheese are allowed in ½-cup servings, and 1-ounce cheese servings, such as string cheese, are an acceptable between-meal snack provided liquid restrictions are followed. Vegetarian animal protein replacement products such as tofu or vegetable and legume patties are acceptable on Day 3.

Measure your portion (1-cup volume or 4 to 6-ounces weight) and eat only until you feel full, not stuffed. If you need to add a moist condiment (mayonnaise, mustard, relish, salsa and the like) to the canned fish I understand, but keep it to a measured serving as indicated on the product label. A universal favorite for Day 3 is the Parmesan Tuna Patties from the recipe section: make it and enjoy! I bet you find this recipe on your menu far beyond the 5DPT. Substitute canned chicken or turkey if you have an allergy or aversion to canned fish.

As a rule on Day 3 fish is the preferred menu option because it is softer and moister than canned poultry. In addition, fish canned in water is considered low fat, a direction we are heading during the 5DPT. However, the chicken and poultry will take on a softer texture when prepared according to the recipes provided and it will work in much the same way as canned fish. And never underestimate the egg dishes and breakfast bakes for any meal on Day 3. These are tasty, economical, and family friendly recipes that are delicious any time and sure to become favorites on Day 6 and beyond. As you advance to Days 4 and 5 you may enjoy any leftovers from your Day 3 recipes.

The 5DPT is a program of advancing our diet following the same dietary progression we were instructed to follow immediately after surgery. That means you can always advance foods from the early stages (Days 1 and 2 for example) to the later stages (Days 3, 4, and 5). If a food was allowed for Days 1 and 2 you can enjoy the same food as part of your menu during the next three days and beyond. For best results meals should be from the menu plan on the day. Snack options may come from the earlier days of the 5DPT.

DAY 3 KEY LEARNING POINTS:

Surrender to change. This is what it takes to survive. Weight loss surgery affects a profound change on the body. Now is your chance to let your mind catch-up and embrace that change.

Practice mental presence.

Rethinking the way we eat. When we learn to work our tool in the real world we are winning the battle. Use the 5DPT as your vehicle to LivingAfterWLS in the real world!

In this age of instant information access we have the advantage of looking online at restaurant menus before ever going out to eat. A little reconnaissance work gives us the power to make informed choices when ordering our meal. There is a triumphant feeling that comes with living in the real world and making our WLS work at the same time.

MY NOTES DAY 3:

BE KIND

We didn't ask for obesity and we didn't ask for the fight of a lifetime to keep it under control. Treat yourself kindly. Find your personal hell-bent determination. You already know how courageous and powerful you are: you learned that when you underwent bariatric surgery. The 5 Day Pouch Test will help you find that place again through the course of five days focused on your mental and physical wellness. Pull out your strength and reserves and let's do this together.

DAY 4- FIRM PROTEINS

By Day 4 the carbohydrate cycle is broken and the liquid restrictions are becoming a habit. Most people report a genuine feeling of pouch-tightness, as they emerge ready to enjoy firm protein. Our Day 4 meals and eating habits are starting to feel like the new normal. And indeed, this is the way we need to eat in order to manage our weight after surgery. Our meals should be Protein First enjoyed with small portions of well-chosen vegetables and fruits. Remember the 2B/1B Rhythm: 2 Bites Protein, 1 Bite Complex Carbohydrate. Take time to chew every bite, resting the fork between bites, and enjoy the meal. Observe the liquid restrictions in order to achieve fullness and benefit from the nutrients in our food. Avoid slider foods and snacking on non-nutritional belly-filler foods. Welcome to Day 4: Today is your new normal.

Day 4 protein recommendations: ground meat (beef, turkey, lamb, game) cooked dry and lightly seasoned; shellfish, scallops, lobster, steamed and seasoned only with lemon; salmon, or halibut steaks, grilled and lightly seasoned. Vegetarian products including tofu and vegetable burgers are acceptable. Be sure to give the Salisbury Steak recipe a try and keep it in your menu rotation well beyond the 5 Day Pouch Test.

By now you should be experiencing that familiar tightness that will assure you that your pouch is working. Remember to drink plenty of water between meals. Take some time to appreciate the power of your pouch. Often we don't like that uncomfortable tightness in the pouch after eating just a few bites of firm protein without liquids. The tightness is reminiscent of a post-Thanksgiving feast that leads to a gluttony-induced nap. It is this tightness that makes the surgery work. And ironically, it is this tightness that leads us unaware back to slider foods, which do not cause discomfort: they sit better and we can prolong the enjoyment of eating.

On Day 4 and forever in your new normal the discomfort in your pouch is the signal to stop eating. This is the new normal. Concentrate today on how your pouch feels and put the fork down at the first sign of fullness. Stop short of the discomfort. This is how the weight loss surgery tool is meant to work. This is how you, the owner of the tool, can optimize the performance of the tool. I hope you are rediscovering your tool and enjoying relief and excitement knowing your pouch still works.

DAY 4 KEY LEARNING POINTS:

This is our new normal: the way we will eat to manage our health and weight with weight loss surgery. The Four Rules are now a way of life and a matter of habit.

Look beyond the breakfast cereal box to feed your body at the beginning of the day.

As recovering morbidly obese people it is important to understand the signals our body sends in order to lose weight and not become morbidly obese again. After all, ignoring these signals contributed to our obesity in the first place.

Feeling hunger is not a moral problem: it is one small part of a very complicated biological process. The 5DPT is a powerful tool and a great step toward building a better relationship with food and your weight loss surgery.

MY NOTES DAY 4:

LEARNING PROCESS

Keep learning. Use the 5 Day Pouch Test and beyond to continue your education about health, nutrition, weight management, and living after weight loss surgery. Continued education works to keep us informed, trying new things, and renewed hope that lasting remission from our medical disorder is achievable. Seek knowledge from reputable publications and from peers. This process of support and learning becomes a self-fulfilling prophecy as we benefit from the give-and-take of a generous spirit. Learn, teach, and share.

We are in this together.

DAY 5 – SOLID PROTEINS

You have made it to Day 5: Congratulations! I hope you are feeling strong and powerful and in charge of your weight loss surgery tool. I knew you could do it and I am proud of you. Today you conclude the test and prepare to embark on Day 6 and the eating plan you will follow consistently to continue losing weight and maintain the healthy weight you desire.

Day 5 Protein Recommendations: On our final day, Day 5, we introduce solid protein back to our menu. Protein Recommendations: white meat poultry cooked dry and lightly seasoned, beefsteak (if tolerated) grilled or broiled, and anything from Day 3 such as the Breakfast Bakes and anything from Day 4.

Remember to chew-chew-chew. Measure your portion and eat only until you feel your pouch tighten. Please, take only 15 minutes per meal and avoid lingering which eventually leads to a grazing habit. By now you should be out of any carb cycle you were in and perhaps you have lost a pound or two. You have renewed confidence in your pouch and your ability to work the tool for your health and emotional wellness. You did not have the surgery in vain: You still have your tool.

Today, do not go hungry. Remember, you can eat as often as you want provided it is solid protein, consumed without liquids and measured in 4 to 6-ounce portions. Be mindful of the hunger signals your body sends as well as the satiation signals it sends. These signals are your ally in the cause of weight management. Day 5 is not the end of the 5 Day Pouch Test: Day 5 is the beginning of treating your body well and managing your health according to the principles of weight loss surgery. This is the exciting beginning of your new and improved living after weight loss surgery! You Have Arrived!

DAY 5 KEY LEARNING POINTS

Losing weight is a matter of health: it is not a competitive sport. Contrary to popular culture, weight loss is not a contest. Weight loss is a lifesaving initiative owned by the one taking action. This is your journey: enjoy it at your pace.

Learn to measure your worth by means other than the bathroom scale. Focus on your whole self: your intelligence, social grace, spiritual connections, and professional and scholastic achievements.

Develop strategies for navigating in the real world. When we have surgery we changed and then we returned to the exact environment we lived in prior to surgery: the very environment that contributed to our obesity. The only chance we have to make the surgery work is to evolve strategies for navigating our new body in the old waters.

Always practice kindness. Be kind to yourself, our ongoing theme. Express gratitude for your weight loss tool and for your personal empowerment. Celebrate doing the best you could to find a middle ground to respect yourself and your traditions and your new WLS body. This you deserve.

TAKE ACTION IF REGAIN HAPPENS

Speak with your bariatric center. According to the American Society of Metabolic and Bariatric Surgeons inadequate weight loss or weight regain should prompt evaluation for (1) surgical failure with loss of integrity of the gastric pouch in gastroplasty or RYGB (2) testing for enlarged GJ stoma diameter, (3) a poorly adjusted gastric band, and (4) development of maladaptive eating behaviors or psychological complications. Find a bariatric center near you at http://asmbs.org/

Honest evaluation. Assess your eating and exercise evolution and return to the lifestyle prescribed at the time of surgery. Use the 5 Day Pouch Test as a mechanism for returning to dietary and lifestyle compliance prescribed at the time of surgery.

Pursue knowledge. Become educated on nutritional health, physical fitness, and spiritual wellness so they may work in harmony to heal your body. Act upon what you learn. Take action. Knowledge is a powerful tool in our pursuit of healthy weight management.

Enlist help. Seek the support of family, friends, community, health care professionals, and fellow patients to help maintain your personal investment and motivation. By the same token: give support. Empowering others is a dynamic exercise in personal motivation.

Weight regain is complicated. Remember, weight regain following WLS is not a simple matter. According to experts, "Weight regain after gastric surgery is multi-factorial and likely involves a complex interplay between a permissive psychosocial environment, nutritional habits, and a complex genetic and anatomic milieu that effect many physiological regulatory pathways controlling food intake behavior and energy metabolism after the procedure." *(Barham K. Abu Dayyeh, 2011)*

MY NOTES DAY 5:

FREQUENTLY ASKED QUESTIONS & ANSWERS

This is a collection of the Frequently Asked Questions and Answers about the 5 Day Pouch Test. Please review them closely as they contain valuable information that will enable you to complete the 5DPT successfully.

Can I repeat the liquid days instead of going to Day 3?

You can repeat the liquid eating plan of the 5DPT Days 1 and 2, but as soon as you do that you are doing a liquid diet; you are not doing the 5 Day Pouch Test. The intent of the 5DPT is to quickly progress through the post-op dietary stages and get us back to the basics of following our weight loss surgery high protein, low carbohydrate diet. People are sometimes tempted to repeat the liquid days because they have recorded a pleasing weight loss on Days 1 and 2. Keep in mind this weight loss is primarily water loss. In order to keep losing weight one needs to follow a high protein diet that elevates the metabolism into high thermic burn: this is when true weight is lost.

Please follow the 5DPT as it is written: it was developed to help you achieve the best results with your weight loss surgery. We tested it numerous times so you don't have to.

I messed up on Day 1. Should I start over to get it perfect?

I have never done the 5DPT perfectly and I do not know anyone who has. Rather than make the five days about perfection make this time about learning. Little mistakes will not stop the world from turning. So forge ahead doing your very best and forgive little mistakes. Learn from each day, review the key learning points and make notes on your 5 Day Pouch Test Journal. Emerge on Day 6 knowing more about yourself and how to work your tool.

You can do this! One of the biggest dietary mistakes we make is thinking we must be totally perfect or totally imperfect. We do not have to manage our plate with an all or nothing strategy: this has never worked for keeping our obesity under control.

How can soups with beans and meat work for a liquid diet?

The 5 Day Pouch Test calls for two days of protein rich liquids. Normally we think of ready-to-drink protein beverages or homemade concoctions using fruit, yogurt and protein powders as dietary liquids. This is quite typical of the early post-op diet prescribed by many surgical weight loss centers. The 5DPT begins with two days of protein liquids in order to baby the pouch, much as we did immediately post-op. In addition, the liquids are useful in breaking a processed carbohydrate snacking habit or slider food addiction.

Can I have sugar free gum or candy on the 5DPT?

Refer to your original post-surgery dietary instructions to see if sugar free gum and candy are recommended for patients with your procedure. Sugar free products are typically made with sugar alcohols that contribute to digestive distress including gas, bloating, and diarrhea. Many bariatric nutritionists discourage patients from including sugar free sweets in the post-WLS diet. Please follow the recommendations of your bariatric team.

Are dairy products okay to use on the 5DPT?

If you can tolerate milk and dairy products include them in your 5DPT and beyond. See the recipe section. Many WLS patients become lactose intolerant so that is why there is always a caution about using milk products. For those who can tolerate dairy, when used in moderation, it can be a healthy part of your diet.

Are yogurts or cottage cheese allowed on Days 1 & 2?

No, cottage cheese and yogurt should not be used as stand-alone menu choices on Days 1 and 2. However, they may be used as ingredients in protein smoothies. You can introduce yogurt and cottage cheese to your diet on Day 3: Soft Protein.

What is wrong with carbonated-caffeinated beverages?

There are a few reasons carbonated-caffeinated beverages are discouraged. First, they have no nutritional value and beverages that contain caffeine can cause dehydration. There is also the theory that for the body to absorb the carbonation bubbles oxygen is released from the blood stream to hook-up with the oxide molecules to be eliminated through the kidneys and urine. When oxygen levels in the blood go down so does our energy level and our metabolism slows. Finally, recent studies suggest the bubbles stretch the pouch outlet causing permanent dilation of the stoma which leads to regaining weight. (Barham K. Abu Dayyeh, 2011) More importantly, carbonated caffeine-containing beverages are void of nutritional value so why put them in our body?

Why do I need to reduce my coffee or caffeine intake?

Studies and opinions regarding caffeine change frequently in the study of health and nutrition. It has long been believed that caffeine is a diuretic or a substance that causes the body to lose fluid and disrupts the body's water balance, which is vital to our digestive, circulatory, and metabolic systems. This can slow weight loss, lead to thirst, fatigue, and weakness. Some believe there is no nutritional value to caffeine and it can be addictive. Those wishing to eliminate or reduce their caffeine intake should do so gradually. Going cold turkey may cause headaches, irritability, nausea, and other symptoms. Doctors say that if you want to reduce the amount of caffeine you consume, slow down gradually to avoid these withdrawal symptoms. Please stay current with your reading regarding caffeine and nutrition and always seek the advice of your health care professional regarding your individual nutritional needs.

Does that mean drinking coffee will defeat the 5DPT?

Coffee will not defeat the 5 Day Pouch Test. But if you are interested in reducing your coffee and/or caffeine intake now is a good time to gradually cut back.

Why is Emergen-C® fizzy drink allowed?

Most bariatric centers discourage patients from having bubbly carbonated beverages after surgery. The carbonation may cause discomfort in the pouch, may cause the pouch to expand temporarily and may cause temporary or lasting injury to the stoma. In addition, consumption of carbonated beverages generally means empty calories that are eaten with non-nutritional snack foods (think of the ubiquitous movie snack of a soda and popcorn). A fizzy vitamin drink mix is bubbly due to the effervescent reaction when the minerals react with the liquid. The fizz is not the result of pressurized carbon dioxide gas being forced into a liquid as is carbonation. Emergen-C® is an approved vitamin and mineral dietary supplement by most bariatric nutritionists. Some patients prefer to allow the effervescent bubbles to dissipate before drinking the vitamin mix. The rapid absorption of vitamins and minerals dissolved in water is an effective means for patients with malabsorption to take vitamin supplements.

When can I have a protein bar?

Protein bars can be included in your diet on Days 3, 4, and 5 of the 5 Day Pouch Test. Be mindful of the liquid restrictions and avoid consuming beverages as you enjoy your protein bar. Many protein bars are dry and cause thirst. We often turn to warm beverages, such as coffee or cocoa, to wash them down. This turns an otherwise healthy protein-smart choice into a slider food and missed opportunity for nutrient absorption.

On Day 3 can I have refried beans?

You can have refried beans on Day 3. They are low-glycemic and protein dense. Be sure and measure your portion; no more than ½-cup. You get 8 grams of protein in ½-cup so try to include another protein source such as an egg for 7 more grams of protein. In fact a great breakfast on Day 3 is the Mock Breakfast Burrito; take a look at the recipe section.

Always be cautious when eating cooked beans or legumes of any kind and measure your portion at no more than ½-cup. It seems the beans tend to expand once mastication occurs and digestion begins. Eating a larger portion of cooked beans or legumes may cause discomfort including gas, bloating, diarrhea, and/or vomiting.

Is Wendy's chili for lunch on Day 3 a good choice?

Wendy's chili is a popular and acceptable choice for Day 3 of the 5DPT. A small serving of Wendy's Chili (about 1 cup – see note above regarding beans and serving size) provides 190 calories with 14 grams protein, 5 grams fiber, 19 grams carbohydrate (again - low GI), and is low in fat. The sodium comes in high at 830mg in the small serving size. That is 36% of the recommended sodium intake of 2,300mg/day. Enjoy this tasty cup of chili in moderation.

Can I have protein shakes on Days 3, 4 and 5?

You can include protein drinks on Days 3 to 5, but only as between meal snacks if you are hungry. It is best to stick with the menu foods, but on the other hand, if you are hungry or "snacky" go for the protein shake. It will raise your metabolism and satiate your hunger. A protein drink counts as a meal so follow the liquid restrictions. Let your body get the full benefit of this protein and vitamin fortified meal by not washing it down with liquids. Also, if you have scheduled a protein drink in your eating plan take your vitamin supplements with it for better digestion and absorption. When in doubt mindfully enjoy a protein drink first before eating any other snack food. Remember this trick! Even beyond the 5DPT a protein drink is always the best first choice for in between meals snack. A protein drink will serve your snacking needs well without derailing your best efforts for healthy weight management after WLS.

Doing the 5DPT caused constipation. Is this normal?

A protein-dense diet naturally contains less dietary fiber than a high-carbohydrate diet. When the body metabolizes protein there is little waste to be eliminated, therefore feelings of constipation result. What you may be experiencing is reduced waste volume instead of constipation. Here are suggestions to help relieve those feelings:

1/2 apple with skin for your mid-morning and mid-afternoon snack

Increase your fluid intake

Include a water-soluble fiber supplement in your daily diet

Add a fish oil capsule to your diet

Drink an herbal tea that contains senna leaf, hibiscus leaf, licorice root, and/or rhubarb root. Look for a specific laxative tea blend.

Prepare one of the Feed the Carb Monster Soups for days 1 & 2 (each 1-cup serving contains 5 grams dietary fiber) and use this soup for a snack on Days 3, 4, and 5.

Keep in mind that a high protein diet simply does not

produce as much waste as a diet high in carbohydrates and fat. Your bathroom patterns are likely to change when following a high protein diet.

Always address concerns about chronic constipation with your bariatric center or general medical care provider.

No Vegetables on the 5DPT? Why?

Vegetables are to be used only as ingredients in meal preparation, such as salsa on grilled fish or the Carb Monster Soups. By restricting vegetables and fruit (complex carbohydrates) during the five days your body is forced to go into high metabolic burn to digest the protein. This should result in weight loss. In addition, restricting complex carbohydrates and eliminating processed carbohydrates helps regulate your blood sugar (glucose) preventing cravings and energy swings.

Vegetables and low-glycemic fruit should be gradually introduced back to the diet on Day 6 and beyond. The focus must always remain on Protein First. A portion-controlled high-protein diet is how we lose weight after a surgical gastric procedure, and that is how we can maintain a healthy weight for the rest of our life.

What are breakfast options on Days 4 and 5?

Traditional breakfast usually means whole grains, dairy and fruit or juice. The focus on a high protein breakfast presents a challenge to our traditional practices. The 5DPT is a good time to look outside of the cereal box for high protein choices. Protein first thing in the morning is a great way to raise our metabolic thermostat because it takes a lot of energy to metabolize protein. More importantly, a breakfast of 70% protein or more will stabilize our blood sugar and prevent hunger cravings. Here are some ideas:

Eggs, leftover tuna patties from Day 3, measured portions of cottage cheese or yogurt, peel-and-eat shrimp, ground beef, chicken, or turkey patties grilled or broiled, each provide ample protein to start the day. And of course, in a pinch, we can always count on protein drinks or meal replacement bars for the first meal of the day.

I'm on Day 4 and only lost 2 pounds What am I doing wrong?

First, please keep in mind the 5 Day Pouch Test is not a cleanse diet or fad diet to hastily lose weight. It is a controlled method of changing dietary habits in an effort to return to the program prescribed at the time of our weight loss surgery. People do lose weight on the plan because of the dietary changes the plan empowers. This weight loss is considered a sweet bonus, not the primary objective. Please use the plan as a means to lasting weight loss and weight management, not just a quick trick to lose weight. And by the way, losing two pounds in four days is nothing to feel sad about! Congratulations! You can do this!

HELP! I am having horrible gas and bloating.

It is quite common for patients of gastric bypass, gastric banding and gastric sleeve weight loss surgery to report an increase in uncomfortable intestinal bloating and the frequent release of foul and offensive gas. Some patients report the problem of gas to be so offensive they suffer chronic embarrassment leading them to isolation. By its nature gastric surgery changes the human digestive process and increases the occurrence of gas. In addition, weight loss surgery patients follow a high protein, low carbohydrate diet which is also known to cause gas. Understanding what causes excessive flatulence is the first step to implementing therapies to reduce the occurrence and offensiveness of this natural body function.

High Protein Diet: Weight loss surgery patients who follow a strict high protein diet frequently report excessive flatulence beyond the 14 releases per day experienced by adults with a healthy digestive tract. In digestion proteins are broken down with the secretion of hydrocholoric acid which allows the activation of pepsin, a protein digesting enzyme. Weight loss surgery patients become deficient in hydrocholoric acid or pancreatin when their intestines are shortened or bypassed with surgery. Therefore the gastric enzymes and acids to facilitate complete digestion are deficient and excessive gas can be produced. A high protein diet, by nature, is a diet low in fiber intake. The absence of adequate fibrous carbohydrates leads to waste material moving too slowly through the large bowel and constipation and flatulence results.

To reduce the occurrence of flatulence associated with a high protein diet stay hydrated by drinking at least 64 ounces of water daily. The water will help to move food along the digestive and intestinal tract preventing the build-up of gas. Eliminate processed meat, cured meat, beans, tofu and soy products from the diet for several days until symptoms of chronic flatulence are reduced.

Sugar Replacers: Weight loss surgery patients are strongly encouraged to eliminate sugar and sweets from their diet. Many people include products labeled "sugar-free" in their diet to satisfy sweet cravings. Sugar-free products use sugar replacers, a term to describe the sugar alcohols such as mannitol, sorbitol, xylitol, maltitol, isomalt, and lactitol, which provide bulk and sweetness to cookies, hard candies, sugarless gums, jams, and jellies. Sugar alcohols evoke a low glycemic response because the body absorbs them slowly making them slow to enter the bloodstream. However, side effects such as gas, abdominal discomfort, and diarrhea, are so extreme that regulations require food labels to state that "excess consumption may have a laxative effect."

To decrease the gas associated with sugar alcohols eliminate or reduce the intake of food containing sugar alcohol. Do not exceed package serving size of sweets made from sugar alcohol.

Therapies to Reduce Offensive Flatulence: The following therapies may be effective in reducing embarrassing and uncomfortable gas and bloating associated with the diet after gastric weight loss surgery

Beano: A few drops help prevent gas formation. Not effective in preventing bloating and gas pain however will prevent gas-passing or flatulence.

Chamomile, ginger and papaya teas: good digestive aides, nerve tonics, and cramp and pain relievers.

Peppermint oil: relieves flatulence and related pain.

My spouse/partner/friend wants to do the 5DPT with me and they have not had the surgery. Is it okay if they do it with me?

It is great to have a supportive spouse or friend and an organic tummy (non-WLS individual) doing the 5DPT will not be harmed. However, they do not have the benefit of pouch restriction and may experience hunger with the portion restrictions. Have them follow the FDA guidelines for serving size and avoid the higher fat soups that could be over-consumed. A note, many non-surgical testers of the 5DPT report that following the liquid restrictions results in less food consumption. Never diminish the value of having a teammate in the 5DPT; welcome all willing participants and embrace their encouragement.

What happens after the 5DPT?

Beginning on Day 6 after the 5DPT we slowly include complex carbohydrate vegetables and fruit in the diet at a ratio of two-thirds protein to one-third complex carbohydrate when measured by volume. We continue to follow the liquid restrictions and avoid slider foods and stay intently focused on the Four Rules. Now that we have recaptured that hell-bent determination that propelled us to have surgery in the first place we use the momentum in our pursuit of a healthy lifestyle and weight management with bariatric surgery.

I did the 5DPT and lost weight, but it didn't stick. Why?

The motivation for doing the 5DPT should always be to get back on track with the WLS dietary guidelines, not to lose weight. That means we take what we learn during the 5 days and apply it to our lifestyle on Day 6 and beyond. If we do the 5DPT simply to knock-off a few pounds and then go back to the very habits that lead to weight regain we will, naturally, regain the weight and then some. When we consented to weight loss surgery we agreed that for the rest of our life we would follow certain dietary guidelines. If we have drifted from the original guidelines the 5DPT can get us back to basics. At that point we must follow the guidelines we agreed to if we wish to sustain weight loss and keep our obesity in remission. Use this as a means to return to following the instructions you were provided by your surgical weight loss center and nutritionist. Go back to doing what worked for you when you were at your best and losing weight or maintaining weight.

What if the 5DPT shows me my pouch is broken?

If you have given the 5DPT your best effort and you still feel like your pouch is not working in the way it was intended to work please see your bariatric surgeon. Several diagnostic tests are available to determine the state of your pouch. In some cases a surgical revision may be necessary due to a pouch failure. Notice it is a pouch failure, not a personal failure when a revision is necessary. Revisions for gastric surgery are common and sadly some needing revisions are made to feel like moral failures when this is not at all the case. A revision is a medical procedure to correct a medical condition. Seek the care of a qualified bariatric team and do what is necessary to protect your health.

How soon can I do the 5DPT again?

Always keep in mind that the 5 Day Pouch Test is to be used a vehicle to get back on track with your WLS basics. It should not be used as a fad diet to quickly knock off a few pounds. Include the 5DPT in your weight management when you do not feel in control of your eating or cravings, when you have strayed from the Four Rules and basic tenets that have worked in the past to help you lose weight, and when you simply need to get back to the basics of WLS. Do the 5DPT when you are in a place mentally to take charge of your health and commit to getting back on track. This gives you the best chance for success. The focus should always be on learning to use the tools that will keep us on track for the long-term.

How much weight can I lose?

The 5 Day Pouch Test is not a plan to lose weight, although many people who do the plan report weight loss. When we reach a point where we need to get back to basics with our weight loss surgery the 5DPT is a tool to quickly get us back on track. Closely following the plan helps us break a slider food snacking habit that may have stalled weight loss or caused weight gain. The 5DPT takes our stomach pouch through the dietary progression we followed after surgery with two days of liquid pampering and three days of advancing from soft protein to firm protein to solid protein. During the five days we focus on the Four Rules, especially Protein First. We observe the liquid restrictions and focus on the very reasons we had weight loss surgery in the first place. Most importantly, the 5 Day Pouch Test gives us a renewed sense of confidence in our surgical pouch and our personal power in following a healthy eating plan that supports weight loss and weight maintenance. Any weight loss is incidental to that and should be considered a bonus, not the foremost objective.

Will the 5DPT work for my procedure?

The 5DPT has been successfully completed by men and women with all surgical procedures. All case studies report returning to the high protein, low carbohydrate diet following completion of the test. Gastric bypass patients report the most noticeable tightness in the surgical gastric pouch and in achieving feelings of fullness more quickly. However, adjustable gastric banding (lap-band) patients and gastric sleeve patients report feeling full sooner after doing the 5DPT. People who have done the 5DPT consistently note that returning to liquid restrictions is the single most important action for optimizing the low-volume capacity of their gastric pouch. Again, if you feel you need to get back to the basics of your post-surgical bariatric diet give the 5DPT a try. It is only five days and you may be surprised how powerful you and your pouch are.

I had surgery many years ago. Is it too late for me?

Only you can answer this question. I know of people who had bariatric surgery back in the 1980's --when the procedure was a simple staple line down the stomach-- who have successfully done the 5DPT. Many times when people ask me if it is too late to do the 5DPT it is out of fear: fear they will learn their pouch no longer works or fear they will learn the pouch does work. The simple back to basics 5DPT will not cause harm and it is only 5 days of your life. So it is up to you to decide if it is too late.

How soon after surgery can I do the 5DPT?

Without exception patients must follow the dietary program directed by their bariatric center for the first year following surgery. No exceptions. I do not recommend or encourage anyone in the first year post-surgery to do the 5DPT. Please, follow the plan your center prescribed specifically for you.

How often can I do the 5DPT?

If a patient is following the program outlined by their center, if they are losing or maintaining weight and feels energized and in control the 5DPT is not needed. It is a specific action to be taken when a patient needs a methodical method for getting back to the basics of post-WLS living. It is not a gimmick or a trick diet; it is a method of taking control when things are out of control. Think of it as your bariatric airbag and hope you never need to use it. But if you do find yourself in peril this airbag is there ready to be deployed.

Can I do the 5DPT Monday-Friday and then take weekends off?

I hope you won't do this. It takes us back to our pre-surgery diet habits and serves no positive purpose. With surgery it is impossible to put-away the tool for the weekend, so why would we put away our good habits for the weekend? Use the 5 Day Pouch Test as it is designed and move forward with an eye on the long-term goal of better health and weight management making the most of your tool, each day, and every day.

Should I take my vitamins when I'm doing the 5DPT?

Yes, please follow the directions from your doctor or bariatric center and take your vitamin and mineral supplements as prescribed. In addition, take your prescription medications as prescribed. If you have difficulty taking pills without food between meals then take them with a few sips of water about 15 minutes after a meal. Alternatively, try taking them with a mid-morning snack of ½ cup cottage cheese or yogurt. This will help buffer them and prevent the nausea some report when taking vitamins on an empty stomach.

What do I do if carb cravings come back after the 5DPT?

Go Green! Including vegetables in our weight loss surgery diet is not only smart nutrition; it honestly helps tame carbohydrate cravings. Vegetables are complex carbohydrates. They deliver nutrients, minerals, and vitamins to our body and affect blood glucose levels naturally. They give us color and crunch and are willing participants in any preparation from raw and dipped to oven roasted and seasoned with herbs and spices. Remember to follow the 2B/1B rhythm: 2 Bites Protein to 1 Bite Carbohydrate (including vegetable carbohydrate) to keep Protein First in your meal plan. Here are some tips from the USDA for preparing vegetables and enjoying them as part of your healthy plate:

Buy fresh vegetables in season. They cost less and are likely to be at their peak flavor.

Stock up on frozen vegetables for quick and easy cooking in the microwave.

Buy vegetables that are easy to prepare. Pick up pre-washed bags of salad greens and add baby carrots or grape tomatoes for a salad in minutes. Buy packages of veggies such as baby carrots or celery sticks for quick snacks.

Use a microwave to quickly "zap" vegetables. White or sweet potatoes can be baked quickly this way.

Vary your veggie choices to keep meals interesting.

Think soup. Soups are perfect year-round for taming the carb-hungry beast within us all.

Should I exercise during the 5 Day Pouch Test?

If you have been exercising regularly continue on your established schedule during the 5 Day Pouch Test but avoid adding extra exertion, particularly during Days 1&2 when your body is adjusting to different dietary nutrition and you may experience feelings of weariness. If regular exercise *has not* been a part of your program use the 5DPT to introduce it slowly into your lifestyle as exercise will support your greater weight management goals.

Science and medicine confirm that the most effective way to heal the body from the ravages of obesity is to exercise. Exercise means moving the body: walking, stretching, bending, inhaling and exhaling. People who successfully maintain their healthy weight exercise daily, not just for weight loss, but for life.

HOW TO INCREASE DAILY ACTIVITY

We are learning that formal exercise is not always the best or only way to add physical activity to our daily routine. In fact, patients are more likely to become physically active when they gently increase their Activities of Daily Living (ADLs) rather than attempt a full-steam-ahead boot camp style cardio and strength training regimen from the get-go. The well-known Duke Diet for healthy and lasting weight loss suggests that the first element of fitness is the ADLs which include everything from "waking up, getting out of bed, combing your hair, putting on your robe, stepping out to get the newspaper to doing household chores, taking care of the yard, and walking the dog." According to the Duke Diet program ADLs accumulate throughout the day and burn calories with little or no conscious effort.

There is never a time following bariatric surgery when it is too late to begin including more motion and activity in our daily routine. Consider these opportunities to increase Activities of Daily Living starting today:

Do moderate housework like vacuuming and sweeping more frequently and more energetically.

During TV commercial breaks stand and walk in place, do stretches, knee bends, or arm circles.

Take the dog for longer, more frequent walks.

Play actively with children and include brisk walking, bending, tossing or climbing movements at the park or playground.

Enthusiastically work in the garden mowing the lawn or raking leaves.

Use stairs instead of elevators or escalators going both up and down.

Take stretching breaks to loosen tight muscles during long working days at a desk or office job.

Stand for routine office tasks like sorting paperwork or filing and talking on the phone.

Do calf raises while standing on line or waiting.

Plan hometown walking tours for a leisurely afternoon and explore your neighborhood.

Bring groceries from the car into the house one bag at a time increasing steps, do arm curls with heavier items such as canned goods before putting away.

Discover your own opportunities to increase your Activities of Daily Living!

A viable goal is to make regular exercise a part of your 5 Day Pouch Test and a regular part of your Day 6 and beyond lifestyle. Include at least 30 minutes of exercise every day on most days of the week. A brisk 15-minute walk following each meal is ideal. Intermittent activity throughout the day will increase metabolism and improve blood oxygenation and circulation. Exercise does wonders for your mood. You do not have to run a marathon or bench press a small child. Simply get up, get going, and get moving. Make it a priority to nurture your health and spirit with movement.

THOUGHTFUL REVIEW:

Gentle reminder: This is not about perfection. I have never done the 5DPT perfectly and I do not know anyone that has. Rather than make the five days about perfection make this time about learning. Little mistakes will not stop the world from turning. So forge ahead doing your very best and forgive little mistakes. Learn from each day, make notes on your 5 Day Pouch Test Journal, and emerge on Day 6 knowing more about yourself and how to work your tool. You can do this!

If we complete the 5 Day Pouch Test having learned a few things about our self, our weight loss surgery and our capability in managing life and weight loss surgery in relationship to one another we have succeeded: we can deem the 5 Day Pouch Test a success. Here are some things to consider while embracing the 5DPT as a learning experience:

What can I eat that gives my pouch a feeling of fullness? What do I eat that fails to give my pouch a feeling of fullness?

Have the liquid restrictions become automatic to me? Do I have heightened awareness of how I consume liquids with my meals and snacks?

Am I eating protein in a ratio of 2 bites protein to 1 bite complex carbohydrate? (2B/1B Rhythm)

Have I found time to include physical activity in my daily routine?

Am I allowing myself to feel empowered when I make choices that nourish my body and respect my weight loss surgery?

Am I forgiving lapses in compliance with my guidelines and moving forward to make better choices the next time?

5 DAY POUCH TEST RECIPES

Included in this Express Study Guide are sample recipes for each day of the 5 Day Pouch Test. You can find more recipes online at 5DayPouchTest.com and the complete collection of tested and proven recipes in the 5 Day Pouch Test Owner's Manual (see Additional Resources at the end of this study guide) and in our LivingAfterWLS Shorts Vol. 2: 5 Day Pouch Test Complete Recipe Collection available in eBook and print.

HELPFUL HINTS:

Avoid substitutions: During the 5DPT please avoid substitutions as much as possible. Each recipe is designed specifically for the designated day of the plan with the amount of protein, carbohydrate, and fat it contains. Changes may decrease the effectiveness of your plan.

Nutritional Analysis: Every effort has been made to check the accuracy of the nutritional information that appears with each recipe. However, because numerous variables account for a wide range of values for certain foods, nutritive analyses in this book should be considered approximate. Different results may be obtained by using different nutrient databases and different brand-name products.

Days 1&2: Choco-Mocha Morning Smoothie

Ingredients:
1 scoop chocolate protein powder
1 cup skim milk or soy milk
1 tablespoon of decaf instant coffee granules
1 Tablespoon DaVinci chocolate sugar free syrup

Directions: Place all ingredients in the blender and blend until smooth and foamy. Hint: If you like an iced smoothie, make ice cubes from brewed coffee and add them to the ingredients as desired. Nutritionals will vary depending upon ingredients and products used. Refer to product label to estimate nutritional values.

Days 1 & 2: High Protein Gelatin

This is the recipe commonly prepared in hospitals for patients recovering from gastric and intestinal surgeries. Many WLS patients continue to include this health-promoting mini-meal in their diet long after healing from surgery.

Ingredients:
1 (4 servings) package sugar free gelatin, any flavor
1/3 cup dried (powdered) egg whites
boiling water and cold water per package directions

Directions: Prepare the sugar-free gelatin according to package directions. When gelatin is dissolved and cold water has been added whisk-in powdered egg whites until completely dissolved. Do not substitute liquid egg whites. Chill until set. Serve cold. For a treat add a 1-tablespoon dollop of fat-free, sugar free non-dairy topping. Nutrition: 4 servings. Per serving: 35 calories, 9 grams protein.

MEASURE SOUP SERVINGS

What I've learned is that soups must be measured. Clear soups or smooth soups without solids should be measured in 1-cup servings and eaten within about 15 minutes. Soups and stews with solids must also be measured, but differently. Use a slotted spoon scoop out solids into a 1/2-cup measuring cup. Put that in your bowl, and then add an additional 1/2-cup of the soup - both liquid and solids. This makes a good hearty 1-cup serving that should keep us full and satiated for a long time after the meal. Thick chili with beans and meat is best measured in 2/3-cup servings. It seems like these hearty dishes are much more filling: it is best to start with a smaller portion. Again, with hearty chili and stews avoid exceeding more than 1-cup volume for any meal.

Days 1&2: Low-Carb Pumpkin & Sausage Soup

This has become an instant favorite for many 5 Day Pouch Test veterans. In place of the pumpkin use a butternut squash puree if you prefer. Canned pumpkin puree is nearly as nutritious as raw pumpkin containing vitamin A, beta carotene and dietary fiber. Pumpkin is a versatile ingredient in soups, casseroles and baked goods that serves our nutritional health well beyond the ubiquitous Thanksgiving pie. Try this soup and keep it in your menu rotation well beyond the 5 Day Pouch Test.

Ingredients:
16 ounces country style sausage*
1 small onion, minced (about ½ cup)
1 clove garlic, minced
1 tablespoon Italian seasoning
1 cup fresh mushrooms, chopped
1 can (15-ounce) pumpkin
5 cups chicken broth, reduced-sodium
½ cup heavy cream
½ cup sour cream
½ cup water

Directions: Over medium heat cook the sausage breaking into small bits. Drain fat. Add the onion, garlic, Italian seasoning, and mushrooms, and cook and stir until vegetables are tender. Add the canned pumpkin, and the broth, stirring well. Cook at a low simmer for 20 to 30 minutes. Remove from heat and stir in heavy cream, sour cream, and water. Serve warm. This soup freezes well in single-serving portions. This soup should not be pureed. Nutrition: Serves 8. Per 1-cup serving: 376 calories, 15 grams protein, 32 grams fat, 9 grams carbohydrate.

Ingredient Note: Country style sausage is bulk ground sausage not in casings. Jimmy Dean® Premium Pork Mild Country Sausage, also called Roll Sausage, is a nationally available country style sausage that works very well in this recipe.

Days 1 & 2: Cream of Turkey Soup

This is a quick and healthy way to use leftover Thanksgiving turkey. Leftover chicken or shredded rotisserie chicken is also good in place of the turkey.

Ingredients:
4 tablespoons (½ stick) unsalted butter
1 large onion, chopped
10 ounces cooked turkey, finely shredded (discard skin)
2½ cups chicken stock
1 tablespoon fresh tarragon
½ cup heavy cream

Directions: Melt the butter in a large, heavy bottom pan, then add the onion and cook for 3 minutes. Add the turkey to the pan with 1½ cups of the chicken stock. Bring to a boil, then let simmer for 20 minutes. Remove the pan from the heat and let cool. Transfer the soup to a food processor or blender and process until smooth. Add the remainder of the stock and season to taste with salt and pepper. Garnish with the tarragon and add a swirl of heavy cream. Serve warm. Nutrition: Serves 4. Per serving: 342 calories, 18 grams protein, 28 grams fat, 4 grams carbohydrate.

Day 3: Mock Breakfast Burrito

Start your morning with this Mock Breakfast Burrito and you will have energy to burn. You may not be able to hold this full serving, so refrigerate leftovers for a snack if you get hungry later in the day

Ingredients:
2 eggs or ½ cup egg substitute
cooking spray
1 ounce Cheddar cheese, shredded
2 tablespoons refried beans
1 tablespoon salsa

Directions: Measure the refried beans onto your plate and heat until warm in microwave. Set aside. Spray an 8-inch skillet with cooking spray and scramble eggs or egg substitute to desired doneness adding cheese in the last minute of cooking. Top heated beans with egg mixture and salsa. Nutrition: Serves 1. Per serving: 174 calories, 13 grams protein, 9 grams fat, 2 grams dietary fiber.

Day 3: Parmesan Tuna Patties

By and far this is the favorite recipe of the 5 Day Pouch Test. In fact, after serving this recipe to the people at your table you can expect to have it requested over and over again. Tuna is an outstanding source of lean protein at 27 grams per 4 ounce serving. Tuna also provides good amounts of healthful omega-3 fatty acids which contribute to healthy circulation and heart health.

Ingredients:
1 (6 ounce) can albacore tuna, in water
1 tablespoon mayonnaise
1 large egg
2 tablespoons Parmesan cheese
2 tablespoons ground flax meal
1 dash each garlic powder, onion powder, salt

Directions: Drain tuna. Blend all ingredients in a medium size bowl and form into patties. Fry in oil (I use olive oil, but you may use cooking spray) until brown on edges. Turn and continue to cook until done. Nutrition: Recipe makes 4 patties. Each tuna patty provides 132 calories, 16 grams protein, 7 grams fat, 2 grams carbohydrate.

Ingredient Note: Flax meal, made of ground flaxseed, is rich in omega-3 fatty acids which appear to help lower the risk of heart disease. Flaxseed adds a mild nutty flavor to foods and should be included regularly in a healthy diet. Weight loss surgery patients should use ground flax meal rather than flaxseed for ease of digestion.

Day 4: Parmesan Baked Fish

This mayonnaise-Parmesan topping is great on baked firm-flesh fish of all kinds. Use frozen fish fillets that have been thawed per package directions, or select the freshest fillet from your fish market on the day the recipe will be prepared. This is a fantastic dish and method to include on your Day 6 and beyond menu.

Ingredients:
¼ cup low-fat mayonnaise or salad dressing
2 tablespoons grated Parmesan cheese
1 tablespoon snipped fresh chives or sliced green onion
1 teaspoon Worcestershire sauce
cooking spray
4 (4 to 6-ounce) fresh or frozen and thawed skinless fish fillets

Directions: Sauce. In a small bowl stir together mayonnaise, Parmesan cheese, chives, and Worcestershire sauce. Set aside. Baked Fish. Preheat oven to 450°F degrees. Rinse fish; pat dry with paper towels. Place fish in a 2-quart square or rectangular baking dish coated with cooking spray. Spread mayonnaise mixture evenly over fish. Bake, uncovered, in preheated oven for 12 to 15-minutes, or until fish flakes easily when tested with a fork. Nutrition: 145 calories, 21 grams protein, 6 grams fat, 1 gram carbohydrate. Nutrition based on average cold-water fish; refer to package labeling for nutritional data specific to your ingredients.

Day 4: Classic Salisbury Steak

Classic comfort food, Salisbury steak is traditionally a ground beef patty flavored with minced onion and seasonings before being fried or broiled. It was named after a 19th-century English physician, Dr. J. H. Salisbury, who recommended that his patients eat plenty of beef for all manner of ailments. Salisbury steak is often served with gravy made from pan drippings. To suit our different tastes this recipe may be prepared with ground beef, pork or white meat poultry.

Ingredients:
1 pound ground meat of your choice
1/3 cup dry breadcrumbs
½ teaspoon salt
¼ teaspoon pepper
1 egg
1 large onion, sliced
1 can (14.5 ounces) condensed beef broth
1 can (4 ounces) mushrooms, drained
cooking spray
2 tablespoons cold water
2 teaspoons cornstarch

Directions: Mix ground meat, breadcrumbs, salt, pepper and egg; shape into four equal size patties. Over medium-high heat, cook patties in 10-inch skillet sprayed with cooking spray. Turn patties occasionally cooking until brown, about 10 to 12 minutes. Remove to a plate and tent loosely with foil to keep warm. Drain excess fat from skillet. Add onion, broth, and mushrooms, cook and stir to bring browned bits up from pan. In a small bowl whisk together water and cornstarch, then whisk cornstarch mixture into onion mixture, still cooking over medium-high heat. Return patties to pan and simmer about 10-minutes until sauce reduces, and meat patties are cooked and tender. Serve meat patties with ¼ cup of sauce per serving. Note: Below nutrition data is provided for ground beef, pork, and white meat poultry: 1 meat patty with ¼ cup sauce.

Per serving using extra lean ground beef: 321 calories, 27 grams protein, 21 grams fat, 6 grams carbohydrate and 1 gram dietary fiber.

Per serving using lean ground pork: 354 calories, 24 grams protein, 25 grams fat, 6 grams carbohydrate and 1 gram dietary fiber.

Per serving using ground white meat poultry: 225 calories, 25 grams protein, 11 grams fat, 6 grams carbohydrate and 1 gram dietary fiber.

Day 5: Mustard Baked Chicken

This is an easy baked dish that is good for cooler evenings. If you prefer use ready-to-cook boneless skinless chicken pieces in place of the bone-in fryer chicken pieces. It may also be prepared in a slow cooker using frozen chicken pieces and cooking on high 2 to 4-hours or low 4 to 6-hours.

Ingredients:
1 (2½ to 3½ lbs.) broiler-fryer chicken, cut up
cooking spray
1/3 cup brown mustard
1 tablespoon cooking oil
1 tablespoon soy sauce, reduced sodium
2 teaspoons heat-stable granular sugar substitute

Directions: Preheat oven to 425°F. If desired, remove skin from chicken. Place chicken in a 3-quart rectangular baking dish coated with cooking spray. Bake in a preheated oven for 15 minutes. Meanwhile, in a small bowl stir together mustard, oil, soy sauce, and sugar substitute. Remove chicken from oven. Generously brush mustard mixture over chicken. Return to oven and continue baking for 25 minutes or until chicken is tender and no longer pink. Baste occasionally with mustard mixture. Serve warm topped with sauce from baking dish. Nutrition: Serves 6. Per serving: 259 calories, 14 grams fat (3 saturated), 409 mg sodium, 4 grams carbohydrate and 29 grams protein.

Beef Tenderloin Steaks with Roasted Red Pepper Sauce

Roasted red peppers bring a smoky flavor to this meal. Peppers are a super source of vitamin C and contain flavonoids that are believed to fight cancer. The sauce brings just enough moisture to the meat to aid chewing and digestion without it becoming a slider food.

Ingredients:
4 (4-ounce) lean beef tenderloin steaks, boneless
1 tablespoon steak seasoning
salt to taste
1 teaspoon olive oil
1 (7-ounce) jar roasted red peppers in water, drained

Directions: Season each steak with steak seasoning and salt to taste. Heat the olive oil in a 10-inch skillet over medium-high heat. When hot cook steaks 4 to 6-minutes per side. While steaks cook place the roasted red peppers in a blender or food processor and blend until smooth. Season the sauce with salt and pepper to taste. Serve warm steaks with a drizzle of the red pepper sauce. Nutrition: Serves 4. Per serving: 188 calories, 25 grams protein, 3 grams carbohydrate.

KAYE BAILEY

Kaye Bailey is an internationally recognized advocate for patients of weight loss surgery, herself a veteran of gastric bypass surgery since 1999. She is the author of the widely acclaimed 5 Day Pouch Test plan, 5 Day Pouch Test Owner's Manual; and Day 6: Beyond the 5 Day Pouch Test; and Cooking with Kaye – Methods to Meals. This plan has helped thousands of gastric surgery patients to get back to basics and manage their weight with surgery. In a kind and heartfelt manner she engages with fellow weight loss surgery patients empowering them to harness their inner strength as they work toward improved health and wellness. Ms. Bailey is the founder and chairman of LivingAfterWLS, LLC: the parent company of the premier websites LivingAfterWLS.com and 5daypouchtest.com.

LivingAfterWLS publications by Kaye Bailey are available from Amazon.com, CreateSpace.com, and other retail outlets.

THE LIVINGAFTERWLS SHORTS SERIES:

Vol. 1: 5 Day Pouch Test Express Study Guide

Vol. 2: 5 Day Pouch Test Complete Recipe Collection

Vol. 3: Protein First. Understanding and Living the First Rule of WLS

Vol. 4: Breakfast Basics of WLS

Printed in Great Britain
by Amazon.co.uk, Ltd.,
Marston Gate.